TITLE

HOW TO REDUCE BELLY FAT

SUBTITLE

THE ULTIMATE GUIDE ON HOW TO REDUCE BELLY FAT.

TABLE OF CONTENTS

Introduction...4

1. Body weight can be traceable to...........................6

2. 15 best ways to reduce belly fat..................................7

3. Better diets to take...13

4. Diets that should be avoided when losing belly weight...................................17

5. Why you should eat protein..18

6. Problems caused by excess fat.....................................19

7. Benefits of losing belly weight...20

8. More things you should know about belly weight...21

9. How belly weight can make you feel...23

10.Conclusion...24

INTRODUCTION

Belly fat is very rampant in the world today because people are ignorant of the effect of it. The effect and the ways to reduce belly fat is what we aim to explain in this article. Belly fat is also known as visceral fat. This can make someone feel so uncomfortable; it can make people feel so tight in their dresses. Some people may look so slim but with excessive fat or obesity. This can result from the kind of food we eat, the lifestyle we live, sleeplessness and lack of exercise. People with belly fat especially in the abdominal region are at a high risk of having diabetes, heart diseases. This can be so challenging because it can make people look terrible and unattractive even to themselves. Some peoples tummy are so big that when you walk pass them, you will turn back to look at them, you might end up falling into a gutter were you are imagining if a man can be pregnant.

Taking a decision on losing belly fat can be beneficial to an individual's health and can extend your life span. At times people die in ignorance, they see belly fat as a normal thing they can manage all through their lives without knowing that it is a disease. Some are so fat that they no longer see the size of their clothes in the market.

In other to know if you have this belly fat, you can measure your belly with a measuring tape. Anything above 35 inches is abnormal both in men and women.

**BODY WEIGHT CAN BE
TRACEABLE TO;**

- **The amount of calories taking each day:** this is one of the major determinate of belly weight. Most of the food we eat contains calories and when taking excessively will result to abnormal weight gain.

- **An individual's age:** weight can also be traced to the age of an individual. Women usually expand as they get older. From their late 20's to latc 30's there body structure begins to change from the young beautiful slim lady to a big woman with a fat waist and a big tummy. Although it depends on the individuals body type. It is also similar in men but not as obvious as it is in women. Men is strictly based on body type.

- **The amount of calories you burn off through exercise:** As you are taking your morning walk, you are removing excesses from your body and this can determine your body weight.

- **Genetics:** it can be transmitted from parents to children. In this case, people have lesser chances of losing weight. But all hope is not lost because you can help yourself retain your normal shape by doing the right thing. Here an individual is fat because the both parents or either of the parents is fat.

- **Hormones**: this can also contribute to an individual's weight.

15 ways to reduce belly fat.

1. **Drink enough water:** Water is very essential to the body. Some people tend to take this fact for granted but it is really helpful. It removes excesses from the body, it also burn calories. Forming the habit of taking a glass of water very early in the morning before eating any

meal will help you lose weight. Drink water as much as you can in a day.

2. **Avoid too much alcohol:** taking too much alcohol is harmful to the body. This can damage some vital organs in the body. Although when taking little can also have some health benefits. Instead of taking crates of beer to show the world that you are an expert in drinking alcohol, minimize it to 2 bottles or one so as to extend your life span on Earth. You are asked not to take excess alcohol shouldn't mean you should go out and start taking 10 bottles of malt or Coca-Cola, please drink responsibly.

3. **Food that contains much protein:** food with high protein content can help control fat. Many people hate taking beans because sometimes it purges the system, but has high health benefits. Examples of food with high protein contents are; milk, nuts, seeds, eggs, fish and many more.

4. **Avoid eating sugary food:** majority of people don't eat food except if it is sugary. The bad news is that sugary food can increase your abdomen and make it look so big. Sugar has fructose that can cause so many diseases in the body such as liver

disease, obesity, and diabetes. When you take much sugar, you overload the liver with fructose which is now stored in the body as fat.

5. A good exercise: constant exercise can help to burn

calories and improve one's health. Exercises such as,

early morning jogging, walks, lifting of weights can help

reduce belly fat. Eating much and exercising little can

be so harmful.

6. Take green tea: green tea can also help control fats, the caffeine in green tea can help boost the body metabolism. Green tea is mixed with large amount of healthy compounds. Taking it regularly can help you enjoy its benefits fully. Examples of green teas are; matcha green tea powder, sencha green tea, genmaicha green tea, Ginger infused green tea and butter tea blend. We also have other types of tea which includes; Black tea, Oolong tea, White tea and Herbal tea. Choose the one that is suitable for you and take three times daily to achieve maximum results.

7. Avoid eating so much carbohydrate food: carbohydrate is one of the major generators of fat. The lesser you take this the better for you. Examples of carbohydrates foods includes; bread, muffins, crackers, noodles, corn and many more.

8. Reduce the intake of fruit juice: reducing the intake of fruit juice will enable you feel better. Fruit juice contains high sugar but lacks fiber. Research shows that drinks like Coca-Cola contain 140 calories and 40 grams of sugar which is approximately 10 teaspoons of sugar. Fruit juice contains Liquid sugar that is not registered in the brain when consumed, and can end up increasing the level of calories in the body. It will be needful to eliminate sugary drinks completely. The label might be somehow convincing but what producers write on the label might not be exactly what is on the inside. If you are addicted to taking fruit juice, I will advise you to learn how to make homemade juice by yourself with fruits.

9. Get enough sleep: getting enough sleep can make you feel better and give you good stature. This does not mean that you should sleep for 24 hours, but at least 5 or 6 hours in a day. People that sleep less tend to have more belly fat than those that sleeps well.

10. Form a habit of eating vegetables: vegetables such as cabbage, lettuce, cucumber, tomatoes are very good for the body. This helps to build the immune system and protect the body against diseases attack. This is better taking fresh.

11. Avoid eating foods that has trans-fats: trans-fat are fat that are added in packaged food, at times added to cooking foods such as margarine. We have natural and artificial trans-fat. Natural trans-fat are formed by bacteria in the belly of sheep, goats and cattle, it can also be gotten from pork meat while artificial trans-fats are formed during hydrogenation: it is a process by which hydrogen is mixed up with vegetable oil to get a semi-solid product. This hydrogenated oil is used for making margarine.

12. Leave a healthy lifestyle: living healthy is the bedrock of having a normal shape. Knowing the right time for everything can help. Some people take their dinner very late at night; this one on its own can increase the belly. Some people have never taken a walk in there whole life, they take a cab everywhere they go. If you can learn to pack your car and take a walk it will help you greatly.

13. Learn to cook with coconut oil: it is necessary to use coconut oil to cook sometimes because It is a natural oil.

14 Reduce stress: stress can increase belly weight by making the adrenal glands to release cortisol which is also called stress hormone. Stress can result from, having too many jobs at hand at once, unhappiness, been unable to reach your goals.

15. Avoid storing urine in the bladder for a long time.

Avoid allowing your bladder to be too full before emptying it. Some people fill so weak to go and empty there bladder when it is full. Know it today that you are creating a lot of problems for yourself. Too much urine in the system often results to weak kidney, so avoid it. This is an additional information.

BETTER DIETS TO TAKE.

- Avocados
- Nuts
- Chili pepper
- Fruits
- Grapefruit
- Beans
- Leafy greens
- Boiled potatoes
- Whole egg

- Salmon

- Coconut oil

Let's see other benefits of eating the foods mentioned above;

AVOCADO

Apart from weight loss, avocado performs other functions such as:

- Maintains healthy cholesterol levels in the body.

- Helps to protect the eyes, thereby improving our vision.

- Help reduces the risk of diabetes and heart diseases.

POTATOES

- Can boost blood sugar control.
- Help the digestive system.
- It contains antioxidants.

GRAPEFRUIT

- It reduces the level of cholesterol.
- It builds up the immune system
- It assists in lowering blood pressure.
- Blood sugar control.

BEANS

- This is a good source of protein
- It maintains the heart.
- Reduces the risk of cancer
- It helps to control ones appetite.

COCONUT OIL

- It is an anti-aging components
- It serves as a salve for wounds and burns.
- Helps in digestion
- It protects the liver against damage.

CHILI PEPPER

- It relieves pain naturally
- Fight against inflammation.
- It boosts the immune system.

- It clears mucus congestion.

NUTS

- Nuts may lower cholesterol

- High in fiber

- It reduces the risk of heart failure.

- It's a source of other nutrients.

LEAFY GREENS

- A natural source of fiber

- It guard the eyes

- It improves your body and defends it against damages from the sun.

- It increases your body metabolism.

Seeing all this benefits should encourage you to make all this foods a part of your diet. It is very important that you know the function of the food you are eating; you cannot be eating your food ignorantly. Ignorant is a disease that is why I found it necessary to tell you the benefits of some of the foods you eat every day.

DIETS THAT SHOULD BE AVOIDED WHEN LOSING BELLY WEIGHT.

- Candy bars
- Fruit juice
- Ice cream
- Coffees that contains high calories
- Alcohol
- Cakes

- Cookies

- French fries

- White bread

- Pizza

- Pastries

Why you should eat protein

Apart from losing belly weight protein are also useful to the body in several ways.

The benefit includes;

- It builds and repair tissues.

- It is also used for making enzymes, hormones in the body.
- It helps in building bones, muscles, skin and blood.
- Protein is a macro-nutrient that is very essential for the body.

Eat protein but not excess of it, there is a saying

and I quote, "that too much of anything is bad".

Some people would want to overfull there belly with food at once. Protein can convert to fat when eating excessively. Eat in a normal way don't overwork your system with food.

PROBLEMS CAUSED BY EXCESS FAT.

- It can lead to premature death
- Type 2 diabetes
- High blood pressure
- Breathing problem
- Heart disease.

If we can take a close look at all these diseases, we will discover that most death is caused by excessive Fat in the system. 90 percent of people that die every year die as a result of one of this disease especially heart problem. To reduce the rate of death, it will be needful to control how you consume fatty foods.

BENEFITS OF LOSING BELLY WEIGHT

If you can take the decision of removing excess fat from your body, it will be beneficial in several ways such as;

1. It will enable you leave a healthy life and extend your life span. Losing belly fat can make you feel good and live a life free from sickness, no breathing problem, heart disease, cancer, diabetes etc.

2. Makes you presentable: having a flat tummy will make you look smart and presentable.

3.A well functional heart: when there is no excess fat in

your system your heart will function properly.

4. Flexibility of the body: a normal shape will make your body flexible and without heaviness. And with a flexible body you can do what some younger people cannot do.

5. Long life: when you are healthy, you will live long. This does not mean living a long life on a sick bed. It is the life style you

live at a younger age that will determine if you will live healthy when you get older. Losing belly weight will help you live a healthy long life.

MORE THINGS YOU SHOULD KNOW ABOUT BELLY FAT.

In most women, fats are parked in their thighs and hips including their belly while in men it is parked on their belly and some in their hip region too and this is very risky. No matter where it is parked excess fat is not good for anybody. Most at times women with fat hips feel excited because it present them very beautiful outwardly not knowing that fats causes more harm than good. Fat in the abdominal region is worse than any fat in other parts of the body.

Large quantity of fat in the body is subcutaneous that is, the part that is beneath the skin. Visceral fat or belly fat is found in between the liver and the intestines and other organs inclusive. It is also stored in the omentum. Omentum is a tissue that covers the intestines, it becomes strong and thick as it absorbs fat. Belly fat is the major cause of so many health problems. Visceral fat is found in between the abdominal organs and in apron tissue known as omentum.

Women's weight increases as the get older more than men.

Researchers at Harvard found out that, visceral fat stores more of retinol-binding protein 4 (RBP4), a molecule that rises insulin resistance, unlike the subcutaneous fat. As the volume of visceral fat raises, the retinol- binding proteins (RBP4) increases. Subcutaneous fat releases molecules that are very useful for the body, hormone leptin inclusive which works by burning fats that are stored in the brain. Subcutaneous fat also produces another hormone called Adiponectin, this assist in protecting the body against diabetes. It does that by regulating the processing of sugar and fat. Visceral fat also produces Adiponectin, but as the volume of fat increases, the level of production reduces.

HOW BELLY WEIGHT CAN MAKE YOU FEEL.

- It will make you feel terrible.
- Uncomfortable
- Unattractive
- Sick
- Abnormal.
- Unpresentable.

CONCLUSION

Beware that health is wealth, and it is when you prevent what will cause a disease that it will flee. Belly fat is one of the things that is predominant in our society today and it is the major cause of health issues. Some people cannot control there throat in eating some of the bad foods they eat in the name of enjoyment without knowing that they are digging an early grave for themselves. Going on diet and watching the way we live our lives will help us enjoy the fullest of our life. It is better to live a long life in good health than Living a long life on a sick bed. What you eat at a young age is what will determine your body condition at a later age. What you eat is what your body will absorb or digest, you can't eat meat and expect your body to digest vegetables. Cultivating the habit of eating a good diet and adequate exercise is very good. Don't say you can't go on diet because you are poor. You can start cultivating some of these vegetables around your house; this can make it affordable for you.

And as a saying goes, "that knowledge is power". Knowing this will help you to know how long you will live on Earth.